South Node Shaman;
Ireland to Scotland in search of the Druid's Cave

South Node Shaman; Ireland to Scotland in search of the Druid's Cave

Shaman Melodie McBride

To order additional copies of this book, contact:
Xlibris
844-714-8691
www.Xlibris.com
Orders@Xlibris.com
797764

CONTENTS

Introduction vii

Chapter 1   A plan takes shape 1
Chapter 2   Over to Ireland 7
Chapter 3   Irelands Sacred Sites.....................................15
Chapter 4   On to Scotland 21
Chapter 5   Gathering Info..28
Chapter 6   A legends influence.......................................33
Chapter 7   The Cave 39
Chapter 8   Art the back to Ireland..................................45
Chapter 9   The Wall 50

Closing...53

INTRODUCTION

This is the first in a series of travel adventures that takes place in sacred and iconic sites around the world. The books are designed to give the reader tools that will aid in their individual journey to recognize areas in their life cycles that are self-sabotaging. One of these methods being able to navigate through association to cultural impact. Relating to how you were raised, where, when, and by whom. I suppose the most challenging issue has been to communicate the benefits of taking care of one's own health. I'm not saying that my experience is the only way but, it is a way.

These writings are based on the knowledge I have received through education and application. My goal is to relay this knowledge in a balanced way, i.e. yin/yang, pro/con, dark/light etc. Though there is the unavoidable programming. The part of self that wants to tell it my way. How the given situation made me feel. How control of the choice would only play out so long before the reinforced energy of the natural universe took over. This didn't happen once or even twice, it continues to this day. It is how cycles work. It is a life process to learn how to recognize what part of the cycle is detrimental and change that through reinforced action. Time and patience really can be exciting and of course rewarding.

The reader can use this through association. We all have different situations we were raised in so not every method will apply. Although there will be something because the energy of synchronicity has brought you here as the reader.

This part of the journey happens after I regained my physical health. Getting your physical body healthy allows your mind state to be in an elevated place and gives you more options to see a situation from a different perspective. I have covered that process in my previous book series 'Going Towards the Nature is Going Towards the Health'.

In my experience the road to cyclic recovery has the most emphasis put on the first year. Which I agree is a critical stage but then what? How do you continue to evolve into a balanced life of your remaking? How do you explain HOW to heal? Or is it recover? Do you really want to recover what led you down the path of abuse? Because the reinforced energy is what moves you into a higher state of mind to see the whole of the situation. Healing would mean the wound is covered, closed. But the scar still remains…then what?

My point is the fact that abuse is there. What you can do, to progress in life, would be to step through with the ability to embrace and accept without drudging the canal deeper. Not only into the abuse received but the abusive behavior learned as a coping mechanism to survive. So use the scars as a means to propel learning in ways that open up positive possibilities for one to live life freely. Thus setting terms to help not hinder the present. Recognition is the key.

This is where I began, by approaching the life cycle from one place of completion and working in reverse. It sounds a bit unorthodox but the bigger view of the entire issue is really the scope of the process. It's about learning to set goals and placing intent in action to achieve them. Seeing the issue in a non-reactive mind state.

You see I believe there is this gullibility that we all carry to a certain degree. This may present itself in any way necessary to the situation, immersing time and space. This leaves the energetic circumstances right for vulnerability. Some of us may know when that is and how it can be used positively, or not, in our lives. While others, such as I, know it will come as chaos ensues. This, is that story.

All in all this is about healing and to realize that in order to have a body maintain its overall health it has to be in flux all the time. Constant influence from all types of energy sources in the 21st century dictate this. The idea is not to ignore it or to put it off for a better time or simply to be able to afford it. Right? So how exactly? It's different for us all. This is my experience and what I've discovered, with the hope others will find tools to aid them on their own path to a more balance life.

Now allow me to explain this book's title 'South Node Shaman'. Why south node? The series is based on my real life adventures toward developing spiritual growth, the second phase after body/mind connection. In my astrological chart my south node is in Capricorn. Adding Astrology in my attention elevated my energy into a higher mind state. It's a tool to aid in developing positive life outcomes. The energy of everything affects the energy of you. What you choose to focus on is what will help or hinder your progress. Being aware of my support and nemesis in the stars has been a great comfort in my own process. Thus, the chaos of the south node for me has authored my life cycles. Of course there are more aspects that influence the chart but what the basics state are that I will follow the hero's journey experiencing unpredictable life expeditions taking me to the brink of chaos to reach divine connection…Every time. I write that with calm but for me its explosive and the learning curve was waaaay steep!

The second query posed is about the Shaman title. Because I research and live many modalities of healing this likens my methods of teaching and writing to the practices of Shamanism. My lineage being from Celtic origin. These practitioners are responsible for maintaining the health and wellbeing of their chosen tribe by learning as many healing methods as possible. Haven chosen this path to help others, writing it down is another means of relaying positive healing energy to those who are drawn to these writings. If I had known this when I set out on these quests you'd think I'd might've changed my mind but nooo, my heart still follows this same course of fate and really I wouldn't' have it any other way.

My trip to emerald isle and velvet highlands happen at the beginning of the eighth year in my recovery with plans unfolding quickly on the back half of the seventh. I state this because to become aware of how ones cycles behave, not only annual but on a multi-yearly basis, supports all aspects of life. The steps revealed to me through the cycles during the first seven years will be covered further on in this series. I wanted to start with the travel due to the different environmental effects of energy that are unknown. You see during the first seven years most, not all, people choose safe places that they know to recover. This was true with me. When you expose yourself to a totally different country stark situations are exposed and it's wise to be on, or in, a place where chaos doesn't destabilize your spirit.

This first journey is based in Ireland and Scotland. Originally I traveled to follow the energy lay lines to the nucleus of northern Europe which happens to converge in the northern hills of Scotland. However, the twist and turns of the Irish knolls and Scottish highlands weave their own tales. The path brought forth ancient stories of a connected history that the Celtic ancestors wanted remembered…and remember I did.

CHAPTER 1

A plan takes shape

NATURE MORPHED THE twisted shadow branches into a dark dragon pasted into the skyline. The mythical image grew from atop the oak grove reaching out to negotiate an embrace. Wanting to touch, to hold, to feel something…anything. It was blackened as though the night had left its presence for the day to hold. My eyes were miles away on a paved road tired from searching the horizon for a sign. A beacon of hope that the direction my companion and I were traveling would lead us to our oasis. Now the dragons ask was met by vision's avenue clearing the journey forward. We would gladly forge the path and follow this mysterious mass.

The day was mostly sunny but cool with an occasional daisy white cloud meandering by in an azure blue sky. It was the kind of day a post card would envy. The Scottish landscape was multifaceted wrapping ones being with the greens of oaks, pines and poplars. The teetering of spring from winter bolstered the colors. The earth rooted pillars are, for me, a connection to everything Nature and the fascinating hidden pockets with fairy coves emerged the more pavement was passed over.

Laden with backpacks full of everything needed for a Gaelic quest, our bodies were aching from the miles upon miles already trodden. Little did we know the miles that lie ahead. This was just the beginning of the unknown paper map pursuit. Time had already presented evidence that energy preservation would be vital.

My cohort Lee was six feet tall with short blond hair, green eyes, high forehead and long neck. Attractive by all standards with an even proportioning between torso and long solid boned legs. These limbs were capped with comfortable hiking boots that had been broken in for the journey. This individual carried a pronounced posture, straightened to protrude strength but with impeccable style. Not afraid of a good days work and loving the outdoors. Hiking was embraced but alternatives would later come to preference as agendas by this individual were revealed. When these green eyes met the end of my index finger pointing out the sign discovered way in the distance the look I received was 'what have you gotten me into now?' Balancing the rhythm of my gait thoughts trailed back to answer the silent question.

It was nine months ago. Energy, interestingly enough, runs cyclic to the needs of the individuals' environmental situation. Creative nature sends a ping out for a response from the universal energetic parameters of like forces. Humans are created in about forty weeks. This cycle permeates throughout our lives of existence. This observation has been clear in my work with others as well as in my own life. Being aware of how energy reinforces progress towards ones goals is a valuable tool.

At that time I was doing research into Celtic Shamanism and the association to earth's energy ley lines. Sites where sacred ceremonies and rituals were held in these areas by the druids was one of my areas of focus. Simply because my lineage had immersed into such rituals and I wanted to know more. I had made simple dowsing rods with hollow wooden handles and bent copper shafts to locate ley lines and was thinking how nice it would be to have a map around the sacred sites in Ireland and Scotland. In addition, I could trace some history of my family since that is where my ancestry lies. Maybe the locations were in close range to each other.

These thoughts culminated one night as I was finishing up a card reading. Sitting on my bed I remembered a book I had ordered a few months back. You know when you buy books that's not essential at the moment but you know the need for it will arise? No? Well I do and I buy books like that all the time only to read later on. Energy that drives me to any knowledge now can be used to associate what future goals may produce. This was one of those times.

I hopped out of bed and went right to the bookshelf where this future knowledge lie pressed and bound. The book was about Ley Lines in northern areas of the United Kingdom and converged energy paths from across northern Europe. It was about to become my constant

　　SHAMAN MELODIE MCBRIDE

companion over several continents. It fell open for me and I began to read. The pages were scribed with sacred geometry, land markers, cupped stones, and hand drawn maps of the areas in my sights. While thumb perusing I discovered the energy nucleus turned out to be in the Scotland highlands. It was made and used by the Druids thus called the 'Druid Cave'. The cavern was placed right on the spot of the main energy source. Wait! (Ah ha moment!) I want to do this! I can do this, I thought.

For the next few minutes I studied the maps and did a bit more research on the area while a plan formed in my head. I had to have a plan to convince Lee to go with me and it had to be good. Now looking back on how this journey came to be in the first place it was actually quite fascinating. As my excitement grew I said out loud 'I want to go!' Lee looked over from the other side of the room and smiled at me. Knowing my enthusiasm gets the best of me sometimes but also aware that when I set my intent, the path opens quickly. This with most likely some sort of associated chaos.

Turning my head to see eye to eye, with a cheeky smile I said 'you know Lee we could go to Ireland and stay with our friends there and see the sacred sites'. The look, solemn but with a one sided upturned mouth and an inquisitive eye twinkle. I closed mouth giggled. Lee had a way of knowing that whatever was in my brain was going to be work but also one hell of an adventure. 'Newgrange and the hill of Tara are close to where are friends live in Bangor'? 'We could even fly over to Glasgow and take a hike in the highlands to look for cupped stones and then hit the museum.' Lee looked right at me with a closed lip half-smile and said 'do you think it's going to be that easy to find the Druid's Cave?' Busted! Smiling back I said; 'I have a plan'! We both laughed and decided to investigate the probability of the trip. Eventually, after agreeing it would be beneficial for us both, it was a go and the process of preparing for a decided thirteen day adventure began. You see Lee is from European lineage and was getting just as excited as I was. In hindsight knowing about my south node life influence would have been helpful at this point. But when you're able and you can, you go.

It was kind of crazy how it fell together so quickly and easily. Lee and I ran a wellness business together and it would have to close for our trip. The schedule would work best over two weekends leaving on a Thursday and back home on a Tuesday with only one full week gone. This worked well for our clients and classes we taught. Closing the business for that long would also mean a financial punch so I made arrangements to have someone there to distribute retail in the middle of the full week gone. That did help offset the cost of the trip somewhat.

Now that the duration and the business were covered it was time to move on to the health travel necessities. This is a vital step for someone who is in the recovery process. What you set as diet has to be addressed at all times no matter where you are or where you go. It is part of the basics you rely on to keep on a balanced level. Going willy-nilly on food and over exuberance is what takes people back into the realm of relapse. This can happen with diet but also sleep and emotional exhaustion. Keeping your base as level as possible when you're going into the unknown will make your adventure much more enjoyable. Plus you will come home refreshed and ready to continue on with the process of cyclic recovery because the benefits of your reinforced choices will be evident. It's really quite exciting.

Spring in Ireland and the UK could be wet and cold so the appropriate hiking gear and back packs had to be taken. We both had a supplement routine that I made packed boxes for and they were placed in the mix. Pretty soon it was decided that a separate box would have to be shipped as we also had protein powder and bars that were routine and couldn't be bought overseas at that time. This was as far as we could go until we spoke with our friends in Ireland.

Mattie and Margret (Maggie) were Lee and I's friends in Ireland. Maggie was from the states and began an online correspondence with Mattie. She had wild dark hair and just as wild of a spirit. Bright with a medium build and a stoic look. She kept emotions close to vest but voiced activation when stirred, especially for the environment. A romantic at heart she loved the Irish brogue in Mattie. He a quiet professor that taught wellness courses in Belfast. Mattie had a not seen in a crowd look. Normal height, short brown hair, clean shaven and could be stirred to reaction with the talk of politics in his homeland. Both in their thirty's and fit, they made a handsome couple.

Maggie had flown over to stay with Mattie and write while they tested their energies in the same space. Independence in the states is much different than in Northern Ireland. This too would be part of the journey for the four of us.

I contacted Maggie and grabbed Lee from the other room as we all sat in on a video session. First I explained to Maggie the ah-ha moment I had and described what we were thinking. She called to Mattie and asked if he wanted some company? Without a missed step the Irish accent came through the mic loud and clear… Aye! So we began to set up the plan.

On my end work and clients had to be taken care of along with rescheduling classes. The planes, hotels, and trains would be a group effort.

The plane out of the US would be via Salt Lake and Newhart into Belfast. We would also need to catch an easy jet flight to Glasgow and back to Belfast. The train would be from Glasgow to Gleneagles and back four days later. The hotel was the Premier Inn Glasgow and Crieff Hydo in Crieff north of Gleneagles. Taxis would be needed at Crieff for a ride out to the trails and back to the train station. Maggie helped set this up so there was an unknown variable to some of the trip.

Maggie was going to send plans for Newgrange, the hill of Tara, and a few surprises that Mattie thought would be fun. These two sites would be visited before we went to Scotland and when we returned Mattie would take us to the Atlantic coast. The schedule was tight but very doable.

In Crieff I will need to locate old maps of the area that had markings to the cave. There is a library in the center of Crieff on Comrie Street that I'll try first. If they don't have what I need then there will be a trip to the tourist information building and I'll go from there.

About a week before leaving we shipped backpacks, vitamin supplements, protein bars, hiking shoes, etc. to Mattie's address so we wouldn't have to pack them on the planes and trains with our luggage.

The box was fifty three pounds and was pricey to ship but there was no way we could've lugged all the extra items with us. Plus it saved us in the long run. Customs thought Mattie was starting a vitamin store. We still laugh about that.

CHAPTER 2

Over to Ireland

EXHAUSTION HAD EVADED the body for adrenaline. I arose with the sun and wouldn't sleep until I was in my seat on the plane for the first leg of the journey out of the US. Details and positive energy ruled the day. The night however would bring a hairline fracture in the energy of progression. Inevitably revealing issues that change brings with the unknown.

We left before midnight only to turn around to pick up my prescription glasses I had left behind. It was a good thing we had given ourselves extra time. Beginning this way the energy was influenced by confounding elements but the overall outcome still remains clouded at this juncture. This is why I journal daily when I travel.

It was a four hour drive to SLC international and we left our ride in the long term parking and grabbed a shuttle that dropped us off at Continental which was the wrong terminal. We walked back to Delta and began to go through the electronic check in but where redirected because we needed 'special handling'. That was the first time I'd been told that at an airport. Apparently we had checked in on the phone but not with the airline. We just shook our heads and played their game so our flight wouldn't be missed. We checked our bags at twenty-six and twenty-seven pounds, were handed our tickets and went to the boarding area to wait.

Once boarded the normal annoyances, such as the person who kept rustling their newspaper and the other who sat next to us and smacked loudly while eating their hummus, could not detour us for the excitement we felt. We were headed to EWR Newark, four hour trip, to change to a Continental flight for our seven hour journey to BFS Belfast. Once in Newark we spoke with an attendant to arrange a seating change so we could sit together and had a spot of time to grab a bite to eat. In the process of walking back to the boarding area a woman came up to me a starred into my eyes. She just stood there and finally asked if we had met. I already knew there was an energetic connection, maybe another life reality, but I didn't know her and stated so. We laughed and she walked away not even exchanging names. I'd been awake more that twenty-four hours at this point and was just going with the flow. There was a precedence being set only to expand as the adventure evolved.

We boarded the Belfast connection and as we settled in for the flight across the Atlantic I noticed a fuel smell. I had experienced this before on long flights and most of the time it dissipated as we leveled at the desired altitude. I covered my mouth and fell asleep. Occasionally startling awake from my own snoring from sheer exhaustion. Lee would've usually giving me a hard time but was also sound asleep. We awoke to eat our vegetarian meal that was served fairly close to our landing time so we stayed awake. Not that ether could've slept being so close to our destination.

The plane began its decent into Belfast. It was a good call to sleep on the flights because rest would avoid us for another twenty-four hours. Fortunately the six hours on the plane would be a life saver for the human condition. I used to believe it was pretty much the same for everyone worldwide, with the exception of some isolated pockets. I grew up to experience that which was part of my family's hand-me-down culture as most do. Lee's story was evident in the 'on edge' energy that was ejected when irritation was felt. I had been engulfed in that energy long enough to know that the unknown would be the captain of that ship. Lee's journey would parallel but not twin my experience.

What was programmed into the culture I stepped into, however, was far different and an open mind had to be my normal. The revolution for Ireland was ebb and flow. The pendulum tends to swing back to civil war. The country's two sides strewn through oppression and famine with religions bias. One land, two views, all Irish opened to invading aggression from outside. There hasn't been a country without two opposing sides when revolution precedes civil conflict. The outcome is

SHAMAN MELODIE MCBRIDE

life for the green and tolerance for the aggressor. Deep chasms remain. The sea surrounds the cliffs of emotions created by ancient mysteries and songs for the lost loved float above the waves into the abyss.

Being surrounded by the sea has an emotional value placed deeply in the Irish. The people take the hardships of the past to build a more secure future. However, the road is long when one tries to forge happiness when paved with grief, famine, and war. Hence, the luck of the Irish is their connection with the land and anywhere this bond is strong others will want to possess it. That being said, I never felt like a stranger. I was welcomed with open arms. It is a place where I feel connected and I appreciate all it has on offer. That feeling began the moment my feet felt the Irish soil. The heart and soul of Ireland.

I think often about the way I felt as I stepped onto the Irish land from the plane. The unknown for me is exciting and chaos is often dialed to the nines. Landing and taxying on the tarmac, the plane stopped to open the door to an outside ramp that led to the ground with a short walk to the terminal door. Excited I stepped onto Belfast and the smell hit me before anything else. It was the aroma of green mixed with fuel from all the modes of transportation around the airport and city. But then the blending began. Like a slide show addition of an old energy. An ancient smell. One that you cannot really see but one you can feel has evolved within the people and culture. Island isolated. Held by the society that for centuries has been invaded from all around. Anxious to be free and, carefree. Knowing that state is not stable. Taking any moment to celebrate ones victories. The people's security in their Island. The lighthouse always watchful for the next invasion from any direction…even from within. Images of faces from the past entered my mind. Not aware of what they know, what role they played or even who they were.

Blending into the crowd the noise from the airport brought my awareness into the present and the magic began with embraces and smiles from Maggie. She was bright with a healthy glow and full of energy. Which, I must say, helped my tiredness extremely well. After picking up our luggage it was on to first a bus and then a train. We chatted about the flight over and what was planned for the day. We came to the conclusion that we had a plan but things could change but at least we had a plan.

Planes, buses and trains were in the agenda for the next ten days and my human condition would be grateful I was wearing a band with a bead in it around my wrist for motion sickness. That little item became my gold gem for the duration of the trip. Saved my hiney is what it did. It kept the pressure on a nerve in my arm, three fingers width south of my wrist, from reaching the 'I have to throw up' center. I wore it every day…everywhere.

This was not the only precautions I took. I made sure I had my vitamins, protein bars for hiking and practiced yoga. I was in my early forties and the discipline was necessary to keep my health in line with the demands of the situations that were to come. Man I was glad I did. I had no idea the endurance a trek like this would require.

As we traveled my thoughts move to the time when my health was not a priority and death was close. My days were pain. I walked, talked, thought and lived in another reality. I had disconnected with me. My body was slung with stretch marks from fat that had wrapped my organs, bones and muscle. Making myself care enough to get up, shower or even eat was exhausting. I was one hundred or more pounds overweight and accepting that I would always be that way was heartbreaking to me. I just couldn't bring my mind in line with that thought so the consequence was to die or get help. It was my programed nature not to ask for help. It meant I was weak. That I couldn't take care of me. The depression was deep and set in heavy like an unmovable stone. It would take three years and so much emotional work I thought I would survive only to go insane. But, fortunately I was trained from a young age to work hard and be independent. This allowed me to survive and be open to others knowledge for the help required to heal. Thoughts trailing into the past helped me realize I can do anything I put my mind to. I am grateful for the taught discipline.

Bringing myself back into the present I enjoyed the scenery as the train clinked along the tracks to Mattie's home. Ireland is as beautiful from the ground as it is from the air. The pace is green. By that I mean there is a balance to life that is allowed to play out in a way not forced.

SHAMAN MELODIE MCBRIDE

I watched the emerald become more pronounced as the misty weather shimmered along the window of sight. My eyes watered along with the drops of life stretching across the glass as I struggled to see it all. Lee was tired so the quiet wasn't surprising but Maggie's silence was deafening. There were hidden energies at play here and I said nothing for I knew revelation takes it's time. Our transport dropped us half a mile from Mattie's home…all up hill.

When we arrived in Bangor Co Down, where Mattie resides, the first order of business was to check the large package that we had sent with our hiking gear and supplements. All arrived in good shape. While Mattie finished up with his new renter in the flat next door we were taken on a brief tour of the home. It was two stories, quaint, well cared for but aged. The main level housed the living area with a seventies furniture layout and wood floor. The bathroom on the main floor consisted of just a sink and toilet. In the kitchen was a small refrigerator/freezer that was the norm for houses in the area because most people ate fresh food. The stove was gas next to the sink with a framed window over it. The clear pane looked out into a small beautiful green backyard with a wooden shed painted to match the back of the house. The pale blue was faded and needed a fresh coat of paint. Upstairs were the bedrooms with one bathroom for the three rooms that had a shower with an instant water heater you had to turn on several minutes before use.

Our room was upstairs with a queen bed which became the area where we organized what would be needed for the coming journey the next few days. I was so excited that I brushed off the ill feeling I had as tired. It wouldn't be long until what was really going on would reveal itself in a voracious way. We repacked for the trip onwards to Mattie's vacation home. Grabbing a quick bite we were out the door once again. Climbing into the back of Mattie's red gumdrop car we drove into a facet of the lime stone isle.

The weather turned cloudy with a mist that was flowing in and out as I watched and listened. Only part of the conversation that my friends were exchanging in reached me. For I was entranced in the adventure. Flowing with the landscape, growing with the green and feeling every movement of the moments. Experiencing no time only what was now. Grateful for this chance.

The city opened into country and soon a cathedral could be seen in the distance. Our first stop Downpatrick and a visit to the Down Cathedral where St Brigid is buried along with St Patrick and St Columba. It was one of the surprises that Mattie had for us and I was thrilled that he had cared so.

There are many legends around the Goddess Bridgette and healing. I felt this deep within my being. Placing this positive energy into the kindness and welfare of all beings represented by the Goddess and Saint brings like experiences into my reality. This leads to doors opening for my education in support of alternative healing methods. I believe this thus it is for me.

The day was still misty and cool. I wore an Irish knit heavy black sweater with denim pants and a purple tie-dye Bohme bag over my shoulder. As I walked up the path to the church I felt a strange draw to the stones on the right side of the front door. The church was closed as it was not yet tourist season so we were alone. I placed my hands on the stones and felt a calming that I enjoyed for a while before I was directed by Maggie to the cemetery. The schedule was tight to get everything in before we flew to Scotland on 11 May. It was now 9 May 2008.

The large stone plate that covered the place where St Brigid was buried had cracked right down the middle and the two halves had falling into each other. I knelt and a sadness overcame me as I held this image in my mind. The other saint's graves were cared for yet this one was left in disarray. Why? I felt the left half and the right with both hands and the tears began to flow. Before I was engulfed in grief Lee pulled me up and said nothing. Looking into my eyes the only thing said was 'it's time to go.' Lee was a very private person emotionally and being such had built huge walls for protection. But Lee felt extreme energy shifts within me and for that, and in that moment, I was grateful.

We took a brief stroll through the field behind the church towards an Abby. It only had a few remaining rock walls that held a partial roof. As we approached the site a bog was revealed that blocked our path from going any further. By now all were cold and wet. We walked back, piled

   SHAMAN MELODIE MCBRIDE

in the gumdrop coach to get warm and finish our journey to Mattie's family home on the east coast.

Newcastle is on the Irish Sea and lies at the base of Slieve Donard. It's a small seaside town in County Down, Northern Ireland with under ten thousand residents. It has a variety of aspects ranging from sandy beaches to forests and mountains. Newcastle has an isolated retirement type feel that draws you into it. Placed into a valley by the sea its golf, hiking, and ocean recreation make it a lovely place to relax.

Once spotted we began our descent. Half hour later we were shopping for groceries so I could prepare dinner for all of us. I had learned to cook in my pre-teens and was very adapt in blending herbs and spices to bring out the flavors in food combinations. This was known by Lee and Maggie and they were all in with me utilizing my culinary skills. You could almost see the watering at the corners of their mouths. Mattie, of course, had been coached by Maggie and was also on board for the experience. After all Ireland was famous for its fresh catch and nutritious vegetables.

We reached Mattie's family home. It had been left to all the siblings and they shared time and cared for the bungalow. It had beautiful large azalea bushes with pink blossoms that smelled heavenly. White with a thatched roof and small yard. Inside there were two bedrooms upstairs with a bath and downstairs one bedroom with half bath. Also on the main level was the kitchen, dining, living room and atrium off the dining area. The atrium was my favorite place although I wouldn't get to experience it until the next morning because it hit. My head exploded and it was so plugged up I couldn't breathe. I lay on the single bed that was one of two in Lee and I's room and put in nose drops to relieve the pressure. Part of me knew this was from the flight as I was inundated with exhaust from the plane but there was more. Something that wouldn't reveal itself until much later.

The next thing I knew Lee was waking me up to fix dinner. Not saying a word but summoning every ounce of any energy I could, I arose and prepared a beautiful feast. At the table after everyone was pleased and plump I took a sip of my tea and awoke the next morning. I don't remember getting up from the table, getting undressed, anything. I was so exhausted but safe. It is understated how important it is to feel safe with the people you're with and the places you stay. Everyone pitched in to help. I felt blessed.

It took me awhile to get myself together the next morning and tea in the atrium assisted my recovery. All were patient and regrouped while waiting. I was weak but not going to miss seeing Newgrange by any means. I optioned out of conversation after we loaded into the gumdrop ride to enlightened dreams and fairy whisperings. The tea and herbs took effect and the day's sunshine did the trick. My health had improved significantly and I felt like I had cleansed away old energy. I knew the door was opening but with this type of beginning, answers would take a high level of endurance and energy. That fact was only encouraging me to go for it!

CHAPTER 3

Irelands Sacred Sites

A VISIT TO IRELAND'S north wouldn't be complete without a stop at the best known passage tomb of Newgrange. It has a beautiful white quartz façade and a large round stone that is covered with engraved spiral patterns in front of the entrance. It is one large tomb. Newgrange is designed to allow light from the winter solstice to enter into the main chamber through a roof box over the only opening. We were all looking forward to visiting the site. Our schedule was tight though because of my illness so it would be the only mound we'd visit although there are several in the area. From Newcastle the tomb was a little over an hour's drive.

Newgrange complex is designed so buses transport you to the tomb and you leave your personal vehicles at the information center. They have each group timed so only one group at a time is on the Newgrange grounds. Fencing also helps enforce the situation. I liked this because I'm not a big fan of mass amounts of people touching my energy.

My health was still in question as we waited in the main lobby. I felt weak and my mind was swimming with thoughts of the past but not mine. We had to wait for a bit so Lee bought me a bottle of water while the two M's toured the information center. I held Lee's arm and slowly joined them. I felt like I had taken on some other type of energy. I didn't know whether it was a trigger from my distant past or someone that maybe I had known. The reality was that it was seriously messing with my psyche and keeping my focus was challenging. That on top of my sinuses still running and constantly wiping my nose. The irritation of it all seemed irrational. I would come to realize the annoyance was not only mine. Lee's anxiety was building in anticipation for part two of the trip.

It began to ease as the view of the tomb grew closer from my window of our bus. When my feet hit the ground a flash of the building of this magnificent structure came to view and again I felt the same presence as when I stepped off the plane in Belfast. I could see the quarry of white stone masons and the bare dirt of the mound. Smoke billowing and skin clothed individuals working as one tribe. I stumbled and Lee caught my arm asking me if I was alright. Assuring Lee I would be fine we continued up the path to the cup marked stone at the entrance of the tomb.

As the group entered the passage the palms of my hands began to heat up from my connection with the healing art I had been attuned to a year earlier. But why? Was this a place of healing in spite of the death that was present? Maybe this is why people feel better when they visit the dead. Maybe it is why people gather today to honor those souls who have passed. So many questions and yet, only perceptive answers.

I smelled the dirt and bone. The odor was so ancient, it was so far away even though I could see the brown of the floor and grey stone walls. Our guide explained the way it is perceived as to the origins of its use. I listened as it was explained about the cupped marked bowl, one of two, that was used for burial ashes but I was in my own thoughts. My own concepts of the energy that was swirling around my being like an invisible dirt devil. The air became thin and I moved away from the group towards the back of the tomb. The guide had seen this and moved us all toward the exit. Our time at the mound was coming to an end.

As we left the inside we stood by the cup marked stone in front of the passage. Our guide instructed the group not to touch it. This after Lee and I had already placed our hands on the stone to feel its energy. Lee and I had been attuned in the ancient healing practice of Reiki several years back and connected to it often when frequencies in energetic patterns were similar to source. It is a practice we used in our business and one I feel often especially around ancient energies. Lee and I then walked around the front with Maggie and Mattie to take in the beautiful white quartz that covered the entire front of the tomb. The sun brightened the stone briefly peeking out of the clouds. I don't know why I gazed directly at the quartz but it white speckled my vision and I could hear the laughter as Mattie guided me back to the path. It was clear I was in a different reality. I was grateful for my comrades. We boarded the bus and headed back to the main center. We had little time to dilly-dally for Maggie and Mattie had a full day planned for us. Back into the gumdrop auto and on to the Hill of Tara around half hour drive south.

We visited Ireland during an off season and Mattie took advantage of this. The Hill of Tara was not crowded with people. As a matter of fact the four of us were the only ones there. This gave us time and presence.

The path began with St. Patricks' Cathedral where stands a statue of the saint before the entrance of the church grounds. We walked into the grave yard and marveled at the skill of the masons, not only for the exquisite little building of worship with its granite corner stones and gothic steeple, but the Celtic knotted crosses used to mark the graves. As we all walked the pairing became different and Lee and Maggie marveled at the ancient trees and grounds of the graveyard.

Mattie and I began to stroll toward Tara discussing Ireland's plight. Stopping briefly because of muddy terrain we gazed at the Lia Fail (Stone of Destiney). The stone sits atop the Hill of Tara and was where the High Kings of Ireland were crowned. The legend says this stone sounded in loud tones for authentic contenders at the coronation.

Walking on we continued our conversation. Mattie spoke of an oppressed happy people sitting on an Emerald Isle tired of being poor. He painted the picture of the decade's old war with Britain, the military foothold they have wanted in Ireland and the people that were born of this land just wanting to be free. Mattie was at peace when speaking of his homeland. Almost a reverence that was part of the process of change. The people of the land still longing for resolution. It brought my mind into a space of contemplation of living in the past. What memories were so traumatic that a culture was affected so deeply? Was it that the perception was always to be of forced adaptation? Or was it just plain old greed from the establishment? All of the fore mentioned, plus so much more, was my understanding in this moment in time. It overwhelmed me with emotion and to my surprise I fought back tears. I suppressed the emotions so I would not interrupt Mattie's flow although I knew he felt my compassion.

We strolled and talked enjoying the beautiful Irish landscape, the sheep with their fluffy tails and watched by the ancient trees that held the memories of children swinging from their strong branches in much happier days. You see this land, the hill of Tara, was in the process of a struggle to be developed and again the people who lived there were having to find their voice once more. To save their cultures historic past.

This also is a reoccurring theme in my life. Where some can shift effortlessly into the event, I am met with chaos. My life swings rapidly into a startled emergence. So am I aware that this venture will also hold this energy. Only to reveal itself whenever it decides the time and energy are right to converge.

As we met up with the two other adventurers at the end of the field Mattie had a surprise for us. He led us to a stone fence and a narrow foot path. As we followed the path down a small hill we rounded the corner to hear water. A small trickling sound and then a well. A sacred well next to the road hidden from view. This was one of Tara's wells. We titled it St Bridge because the majority, including our own, gifts represented the Goddess Saint. It was evident that the locals knew of the wells existence for the offerings ranged from statues to semi-precious stones to small flower arrangements. The water was so clear, pure in sense and we all knelt and gave positive blessings. Presenting a small kyanite stone, (psychic abilities, connecting with Nature, past live recall, empathy), I stretched to lay it inside the small cove above the opening. We filled our containers to quench a thirst for the remainder of our trip.

With the gumdrop ride sparkling from the misty rain we headed back to Bangor. Along the way we would stop and grab a sandwich by the sea. Originally Mattie wanted to take us to the Giant's Causeway but there was a huge cycling tournament happening along the eastern coast and traffic would be rerouted. Having time to relax and have a nice dinner was what the universe ordered. I felt much better. My energy was feeling a bit unpredictable though. This was normal due to the unknown world we were about to enter. Lee had anxiety. Why would be revealed soon enough. Lee was aware of the chaos the shifts

    SHAMAN MELODIE MCBRIDE

in my energy could bring. What would be the sign? Time would tell but in the meantime a good night's rest would foster the quest onward.

The next day we slept in a little and arose to start packing for the next leg of our excursion. I felt really good after the day prior. Although the experience so far was soul enriching, what we were about to encounter could not have played a bigger role in the development of our group as individuals. The separation of energies was about to unfold.

Our flights were in the afternoon so we headed to the beach for a few hours. But first ice cream for Mattie's sweet tooth. I was feeling much better and decided to pass on the sweet treat. Instead I took the opportunity to talk with an older Irish man outside the pearly white shop who was seated at the table next to me.

The man looked the part of a storybook quaint town Irish gentleman with his tweed cap, corded jacket and plaid buttoned vest. Our eyes met and he smiled and tipped his hat as he sipped his drink. He had kind eyes and a nice energy so I wasn't really thinking about what would happen. I just wanted to chat with this man on a sunny day in front of a lovely place in Ireland. I asked about the area and why he lived there. With a bit of hesitation he said 'where else would I live? This is where the lineage of my family sacrificed to settle. Taint leavin it now nor never!' I nodded in agreement. 'Why ya wondering?' he asked. Without a beat, smiling I said 'searching for fairies and druids'. Looking me in the eye his blue pools sparkling said 'better be saying it straight. There be ears in every nook and eyes in all the rounds'. We smiled and then I heard my party coming out the door. I turned in my chair to wave them down. When I turned back around the man was gone. I looked around but he was nowhere. Maggie asked if I was talking to someone because she could hear me as they walked out the door. 'No' I said 'just thinking out loud'. The moment was precious, not to be explained and all mine.

It was mid-May so it was a bit chilly by the sea even though the sun hung in a pale blue sky. The day was relaxing as is the Ireland way. We collected glass off the white sands while watching the children and dogs play on the beach. While mustering up the bravery to take off our shoes and wade in the wake. Man that water was cold! All part of the experience of being in the moment.

The cyclic triggering in the cells causing my illness of the first few days ran in my thoughts. The mind interprets what it needs to fulfill the sense driven cravings. This includes all energy that makes up all the cells throughout the body. It's easy to believe that we are separate, apart from the universe until some profound experience shifts your reality. This new understanding brings you into the awareness of your true connection. You are energy of the universe. Just because your mind has evolved in its time space dimension doesn't mean you don't carry all energy all cells have carried from the beginning. The worst of the cleansing had passed and I was ready for the next leg of journey.

Mattie had a business meeting in Glasgow so he would be boarding with Lee and me while Maggie had a meeting in Dublin. She had originally planned to accompany us to Scotland but had to try and renew her visa for another three months.

Making our way to the airport, Maggie and Mattie only had carry-ons while Lee and I had thirty-five pond backpacks to deal with. But all went well and on touch down we made a plan to meet Mattie at weeks end to fly back to Ireland. Scotland here we come.

     SHAMAN MELODIE MCBRIDE

CHAPTER 4

On to Scotland

IT WAS A quick flight across the pond and after landing Mattie, Lee and I grabbed a taxi to the Premiere hotel on the corner of Argyle Street and James Watt Street in Glasgow. We would attempt to get dinner but just managed a cup of tea with Mattie before he left to prepare for his meeting the following day. We dropped our belongings off in the room checking to make sure it was all good. Then we went out and walked to the Tesco around the corner to grab some snacks and water for the next day. Later we ate at the Thyme restaurant inside the hotel. The meal was good and full of protein for the following days of hiking for Lee and me. Mattie's meal was lighter than ours and after we all enjoyed a sweet treat with an espresso. While conversing with Mattie it become clear what he had assigned his role to be while speaking with us. He became our historian of Irish culture. Being it progressive or lack of, Mattie would prove to be the instrument of knowledge that was ingrained in Northern Ireland's struggles and conquests. We would be all ears once we returned back to Ireland in a few days. But for now it was clear we had a lot of work to do in a very short amount of time.

I must say that Lee had been very supportive of this sacred quest that I created. That support was about to be tested to the nines. Lee checked in with home from the room. The business was fine and Lee's ex-partner was caring for their child. I was only allowed a little bit into this part of Lee's life and that was fine with all involved. It worked out well.

I was busy searching for businesses around our hotel in Crieff for supplies and maps. We had booked another night at the Premier Hotel in Glasgow in three days. The search for the Druid's cave was going to be a lot of work and a bunch of luck. The train and transport to the

Crieff hotel was taken care of by Maggie. She had booked all that and sent us the info via email.

Arising early we made our way to the train station. It was only about a five minute trek. It was forty-nine minutes by train from Glasgow to Gleneagles. The two of us were super excited. We talked about the plan we would make once we arrived in Crieff. The area was chosen because it was closest to the mountain range where the supposed cave resides. When we arrived and stood in the station, a situation became alarmingly clear. The station was unmanned. A detail that had bypassed everyone's awareness and one that would now cause us to put on our thirty pound back packs and start walking.

It was about fifty degrees and we were well dressed so away we went. We had walked half a mile out of our way because we were looking for some kind of bus stop or taxi. We had cell phones but no signal. We found a schedule that stated the wait for a bus would be two hours so we began to walk towards the overpass. We found an officer there at the top stopping traffic so he could guide through an oversized long load truck. He stated that Crieff was eleven miles away but that it was alright to hitchhike and that the road was safe. Lee was not happy. I on the other hand just looked at it as part of the journey that was unfolding into work.

I've always known for me that it just was this way and as long as I went with the flow and kept it positive, things would work out for the greater good. Lee just needed some time which I was more than willing to give. After all that's what you do with someone you love.

As we walked along the paved road toward Crieff, my thoughts wandered back to when I met Lee four years ago. It was one of those moments the French call le flash. Our eyes met and everything changed. I was hired to work for Lee. I did some remodeling and odd jobs while the energy between us grew. Lee was married and I didn't want to cause any problems but in hindsight the meeting of souls was the chaos that the universe planned for all involved. It wasn't long before we had fallen in love but I couldn't continue to be a part of a deceptive pain, so I walked away. Lee had a choice to make alone, without my interference and I would respect that choice. Needless to say the decision

 SHAMAN MELODIE MCBRIDE

was divorce. One year later when all was settled Lee and I were married. A beautiful tropical island wedding. We were so happy, but isn't that how it's supposed to be? There was so much passion. I knew that our life together would be intense after all we connected through the windows of the soul.

Those eyes, those starry, longing, hints of love
They look away in the instant of clarity
Connection with like divines withheld for an illusion longer
Gratitude… The glance lasting to the depth of the heart
Shaman Melodie McBride

Bringing my attention back into the moment was Lee pointing out some ruins and what appeared to be a fairy grove circled by tall old trees. The energy for me was not unlike when I entered Newgrange, wise and so sacred. Although this was Scotland the feeling in the land was like Ireland but not the same. Although the energy within me felt little difference. Nature had supported a community and they had placed a value on respecting the environment for its bounty and the diversity in its destruction and rebirth.

We finished walking around the ruins and hopped back on road A823. Around the next mound of bushes opened up to the back part of the Gleneagles golf course and a slew of noisy birds. As we approached them we noticed the red curved bills and legs with silky black bodies. They were Choughs, pronounced (Chef), and they were so busy eating and socializing there was not a stir among them as we walked by. They hardly noticed us at all.

The sun was nice and as we approached The Gleneagles Golf Course entrance sign and Lee wanted a picture to show people at home so of course I obliged. It was where they held the Rider's Cup you know, very prestigious. You see Lee had a way of completely blocking out what wasn't 'socially right', and often told me what I was thinking and how I felt. This was something that was somewhat of a sore spot for me because it invalidated who I am. So far love had allowed me to overlook this feature of Lee but for how long? The evolution in healing would have it's say in time. For the moment I would do what I must to keep the peace. This was my choice and keeping the energy positive was vital for a spiritual flow in this journey.

The trek was full of small talk about the beautiful scenery and the agenda that we would need to keep on track to find the cave. I couldn't help noticing how the frustration in Lee kept growing. The energy that was being thrown my way caused me to go into my shell to protect myself. This was the way I learned to handle abusive situations now. Before I would just explode and that amounted to a beating as a child more than once. At one point in Lee and I's relationship there was a breaking open point for me that I just screamed out how I didn't know why I was angry. That was a big turning point for me and Lee helped me through it with kindness and understanding. Lee could relate because of the endured abuse that was felt through an upbringing of abusive parents. All in all abused people learn to cope by becoming abusive themselves. This behavior was measured by the abuse applied and the personality of the individual involved. Realizing this, plus taking accountability for my actions, helped me work through the emotional dis-function that led to the self-sabotaging behavior sacrificing my health and wellbeing. I was now forty-five years old and had been working to gain my stability in mind and body for almost a decade, still feeling like a novice. I had so much further to go and with that I was snapped back into reality by Lee wanting to stop at a small farm to fill our water jugs.

Ambling up to a gated pasture a man saw us and came walking towards us with a stern look on his face. I said good day and told him we were going to Crieff and wondered if we could fill our water bottles. He just stood there and looked at us as if we were criminals. Lee said we were staying at the motel in Crieff and wondered if the farmer knew of transportation to get us the rest of the way. 'NO!' he said, 'there's the hose'. We both took a step back as his wife came out and calmed things down. By this time Lee and I had begun to fill our bottles and were doing our best not to be confrontational but Lee couldn't stand it. The farmer's wife listened calmly as Lee barreled into the whole respect your fellow human being speech. I finished filling my jug and eased

      SHAMAN MELODIE MCBRIDE

toward the road thanking them for the water. Lee followed aggravated and tired. I was quiet once again.

I thought about how in Ireland we were treated with kindness and wondered what had happened in this small area of the highlands to cause such aggression. Feeling I could calm Lee I made a statement about just that. "I wonder what happened to that farmer that he would be so hostile. It must have been pretty bad. I'm going to send him healing energy." Lee's expression softened. Nodding, Lee also sent positive energy. We smiled at each other and made a plan to stop soon for a snack now we had water.

About two miles further we found this lovely cove of trees with a large fallen dead log to sit on. We made our way through the grass and sat down to enjoy a protein bar and apple. The sun was so nice and felt so good on my shoulders that had been backpack ridden. In the quiet we sat, ate and then stretched our bodies before donning our packs again. We felt better and our spirits were lifted as we continued down the A823.

I want to interject here my learned experience regarding triggers and playing into them concerning people in our lives we often deal with. When one trigger plays off another because the individuals are in the same energy the realization of wanting to change is brought into the afterthought moment. But because of programmed perception, genetics, recognition of souls maybe from past existences, etc. the person may not be in the awareness of how to change the situation. Or even fully aware how to counter the right and/or wrong in the behavior. Becoming vulnerable is part of trust that tends to be buried into self when chided into being made fun of by one you love. Triggers can come from anywhere. The energy any human being carries comes from many sources in the DNA. Most energies we carry will never be known to us and thus not triggered. The best way I have found to pull out triggers is the unknown. Place a being into a situation that is jarring, weather positive or not, and odds are the means this individuals energy has associate with the event will service. It's okay to be accountable for your own actions and reactions. That's how we learn to evolve as human beings. Self-examination is necessary for one to overcome these triggers in whatever form they manifest. After all where would we be without evolution?

As I continue to ask the universe the question on how to recognize my own triggers I knew the answers would unfold in a matter of time. I must be the one to open up and allow the answer and that, my friends, is a compassion for self that many of us only see glimpses of for short periods of time. For me I would have to drop myself in unknown situations. Chaos is about to unfold and I can see the steps but can I make a better choice? At the end of the day it's about choices we make.

'That's it!' Lee exclaimed 'I've had enough' as I was snapped back into reality. I looked over and Lee's thumb was out trying to hitch a ride. I watched as first one car then another flew by us. Then the third car slowed down and rolled down the window. It was a women in her forties and she looked right at Lee and screamed 'get a job!' That was all it took for the thumb to come in and not go back out again. Now I wouldn't say Lee's a stuffed shirt but pretty close and I just couldn't hold the laughter back. It burst out of me and to Lee's credit a smile appeared on a wounded face. Ego busted, all both of us could do was laugh.

A bit further down the road we came to the end of A823 and turned toward Muthill on A822. It was another two and a half miles according to the sign and we were energized in the progress we had made. Rounding the first corner off in the distance, towards the North a sign on top of the trees.

'Hey!' Lee had brought my awareness back into the present. I smiled and said I was reminiscing over our adventure so far, Lee's face glowed but the eyes were tired. Even though our bodies felt the hike the scenery lifted our feet on again like a soft drumbeat as we used the dark dragon on the treetops as our guide. The sun was shining and we enjoyed the rest of the hike into town.

Entering Muthill we were exhausted. Muthill, meaning 'soft ground', was a small village in Perth and Kinross, Perthshire, Scotland. It sits three miles south of Crieff. We walked to the general store that was painted red. Inside we found some sugar free rocks stars, our favorite, and asked the man for some taxi info. He acted put off about it and sent us to a phone booth down the street that didn't work.

          SHAMAN MELODIE MCBRIDE

Frustrated, we went to the bus stop and decided to wait. I know three miles didn't sound like much but we had just hiked eleven miles with heavy backpacks. We could do it but we were going to look for other means of travel first. This and placing a lot of positive energy calmly into the situation. We were there only about fifteen minutes when a local man asked us where we were headed. I told him we were going to the Crieff Hydo and he stated he was headed close to there to walk his dog. Then he asked us if we'd like a ride. Before I could say anything Lee popped up and said 'YES' and was halfway across the street before I could even grab my backpack. The ride was pleasant and we found out the man was a local artist. It was the first nice person we had met along the road other than the officer.

After unloading and thanking the artist for our salvation ride. We walked into the main lobby of the Crieff Hydo with backpacks and felt quite out of place. It was beautiful. The architecture was stunning. Since 1868 the nine-hundred acre four star hotel founded by Dr. Thomas Henry Meikle is one of the most complete overall resorts in the world. Our reservations were good and all checked in we made our way up the hill to our self-catered two bedroom cabin with kitchen and shower. We dropped off our gear and headed back down to town to pick up some groceries. It was a short walk and all seemed a blur. We found the first market we could, bought dinner for one night and went back to the cabin. I cooked diner while Lee made the beds. We ate and then I fell asleep looking at places that might have maps in town of the surrounding area. Surprisingly finding maps was going to be the biggest obstacle we faced. Lee led me to bed.

CHAPTER 5

Gathering Info

WAKING THE NEXT morning refreshed we doctored our feet with band aids and Reiki. Now full of energy we had a protein shake with our supplements and were off to town. Walking away from the cabin I turned around to take a good look at our accommodations since I was too tired to notice before. It was nice. It was two stories, white with shingled roof and had a cute deck with two chairs by the front door and a deck off the upstairs bedroom. There were other cabins on our lane but all we spaced for privacy and the trees that surrounded all were tall pines. It smelled so wonderfully refreshing. I took a deep breath and strolled down a pine needle path with Lee to our destination…food and maps. I had eating protein bars, nuts, and apples and wanted something more substantial to fuel my body.

When I visit other areas in the world I look for places where I can get food that is synonymous with my diet. I would prefer to shop, prepare and cook food for myself. Lee was on board with this because I am a good chef. The past year I had been taking private Ashtanga yoga lessons that also taught Ayurveda and how to eat for your body type. I was not vegetarian at this point but was working and studying towards that philosophy. Through my research I realized that changing to a vegetarian diet had to be taken slowly and monitored as not to place the body in trauma mode. This would cause the body to store or to shed mass toxins. By working slowly the negative effects in the situation could be minimized. I had been working on this now for almost nine years and every healing modality took me closer to understanding the addictive behavior that led to my poor health and weight gain in the first place. To this day I had lost one hundred and twenty-seven pounds but the emotional and mental work was what was keeping me healthy.

Plus, my weight stayed regulated barely fluctuating more than a few pounds. One of the most important aspects of this process was to keep regular meals times.

The path down to town was lined by old stone apartments, houses, and a private school. There were flowers and nick knack garden features plus loads of plants. The areas streets were clean with few people to be seen. It was the off season for tourists which was enjoyable. I tend to be a focused individual when I have a goal and dealing with a lot of people scatters ones energy. Although my energy tended to be quite pronounced when enacting a plan and sometimes put people off.

We came upon a grocery store that was small with fresh vegetable outside. We picked out some asparagus and fresh cooking herbs then heading inside where we bought condiment items. We were being watched closely by the attendant and even when we paid there was an irritation with us. Something I still don't understand today. Was it because we were in hiking gear? I don't know but when we went into the butcher shop down the road it was the same. I picked out some fresh scallops, which were wrapped up without being cleaned, we paid and picked up the pace back to our cabin.

I don't know what others issues are and I do try to see the situation from all sides but ultimately you can never know what others have perceived or dealt with. What was taught to me was to discern by behavior and action. This method works well except when you don't take your own actions into account in the given situation. So I played a role in how I was being treated. Previously I had judged others on their abusive, immoral, even unlawful behavior. The realization that my life was filled with poor choices, brought about by my reinforcement and customized development of my addictions, would escape my conscious view for years. The fear of acknowledging them in my mind would have brought awareness of my life being ruined with no way back. This is how engrained my programming was and still is to some degree. The key is not to internalize others negative or manipulative opinions. I'm still working on that daily...but aren't we all. Owning your choices comes with rewards from both sides of the fence.

The kitchen in our cabin came stocked with cooking and dining ware. I enjoy cooking. I started when I was twelve years of age and learned from my mother. She taught me the basics and within six months I was preparing dinner for our family of five on Saturdays. I had to plan the meals and my mother chose the recipe I was to follow. It was fun to bond with mom this way as she worked a lot and we only spent time together on the weekends. Being older now my understanding of my mother's stress during my youth has tightened our relationship. I adore my mother.

It was a Tuesday and our train back to Glasgow was set for Thursday. I took a breath and brought myself back in the moment. Staying present was important for me. I proceeded to do the work to make a plan. This calmed me and looking at Lee I asked if everything was set for the walk back to town. The reply was a warming smile and astounding 'you bet'!

We headed over to the bookstore on Main Street. I wanted to find maps of the area that showed the surrounding mountain paths. Walking in we were met by a nice person asking what help we needed. I stated I was looking for maps of the area mountains that had marked trails. The attendant stated that what we were looking for might be found in older maps at the library outside of town. So we bought what they had and headed to the tourist info center to obtain information on taxi services. Maps were on the brain. Once we had figured out the taxi service we called and were dropped off at the library outside town.

The Innerpeffray Library was the first lending library in Scotland. It is located in the hamlet of Innerpeffray, by the River Earn in Perth and Kinross, four miles southeast of Crieff. Robert Hay Drummond, commissioned the construction of the present library building and it opened in 1762. It was closed, disappointed, we walked on a path along the side of the backyard of the library that led us to a cemetery. The door to the tomb was unlocked. I looked at Lee and said 'we need to ask permission to go in'. When we looked over towards the library there was a person in the backyard.

Lee went up to the main house and spoke with one of the curators that was sitting at a table in the backyard. I joined them, introduced myself, and explained why we were there and that our goal was to

     SHAMAN MELODIE MCBRIDE

find a map to direct us to the Druid's cave. Before long the three of us were chatting about ley lines. We were joined by the other curator and then by the governor of the neighborhood. Tea was brought out with a cookie and pretty soon there were maps strewn all over the table and the discussion was on full throttle. I was enthralled in finding the area of the cave while Lee was talking with the governor. The man that was helping me was also into the dynamic of the legend of the cave and excitedly ran back and forth with books and maps.

Unaware of the name 'Druid's Cave' he did state he may know what I was talking about but that he knew it as the bandits cave. This because a thief had used the cave to hide in years past. We located the general area on several beautiful old maps. They were a work of art. The symbols and legends were hand drawn and reflected a bygone era. Associating the general area on the maps we had purchased in town I placed a circle of the area we would hike. It had been several hours of lovely conversation and research. Thanking all we climbed into the taxi and waved good-bye. Things were starting to flow in the right direction.

With maps in hand we headed back to our lodgings. I made us a nice dinner and sat down to map out our path for the next day. No matter what happened the energy was flowing positively for success in completing the spiritual quest that the highlands of Scotland had on offer.

I want to give gratitude here for maps and interject the reality during this time. It was May of 2008 and cell phones were in their infancy. I had a Blackberry cell phone but it had limited memory for photos let alone maps. I had been taught how to read a map when I was a pre-teen. The religion I was involved with throughout my youth and teen years taught how to survive in the mountains. At the highest level of the program you had to hike twelve miles into the campsite over a twenty-four hour period. It was a small group and we spent the night on the ground and learned how to forage and read the stars. This proved invaluable throughout my life but especially now as the highlands were calling.

The maps we had had cup marked stones along the path and that gave me a perfect starting place. There was a large cup marked boulder in a field just off A470 just before Ferntower. We would have a taxi drop us there in the morning. On further reflection it was apparent that we needed one more day to find the cave as a full day was taken up for research. I called the front desk of the hotel and made arrangements to stay another night giving us two more days. We were lucky their seasonal start was a couple weeks away. Meanwhile Lee was calling Mattie to let him know and discovered that he would also be an extra day. Fortuitous. Mattie would inform Maggie who was still in Dublin. I then checked the train schedule and all was set. It was flowing smoothly which meant the energy of the universe supported the change. A sigh of relief fell over me.

As for the rest of the evening Lee had a different idea and the look of love was an invite to turn in early. Upstairs there were two single beds that Lee pushed together. The kissing began. I love the kissing connection to the senses. The passion between Lee and I was almost overwhelming. The touching, breathing and gentle caressing lifted me into a different reality. Everything in me came alive as we were entangled in ecstasy. Waves of energy loving over and over again until the climax twinned. We lay in each other's arms for the night until the dawn warmed the room.

How do you love the butterfly but in moment of sight
The velvet love that floats with the gentle wing beat in my heart
Love has found me and leaves the still silent impression of grace
Delicate butterfly embeds in my soul no loss but gratitude
Shaman Melodie McBride

CHAPTER 6

A legends influence

THE MORNING WAS brisk but sunny and the wind was making the 50°F feel more like forty. Still we bundled up, called a taxi, grabbed our backpacks and were out the door. The driver of the taxi had been the same for a couple rides now and was helping us with info the best he could. He made sure we knew where the signal to our cell phones would be the best in case we ended up lost and needed a ride. It's apparent the areas people were starting to trust us a bit more.

We were dropped at the Foulford Inn. According to the book on ley lines we could follow the trail from the large cup marked stone in the middle of the field on the farm. I was a bit disoriented and led Lee half mile in the wrong direction until I made it to the top of a hill and got us turned around to head in the right direction. This was accomplished because I saw a cupped marked boulder in the field that was the landmark we were searching for. We took pictures by the stone of each other all bundled up in the cold breeze that was humid and bone chilling. The best thing was to keep moving for the days forecast was for sunshine.

We had been walking and hiking now for two days at an average rate of ten to twelve miles a day, not to mention the time in Ireland. The cold was wearing on our moods but the scenery was astounding. I'm a tree hugger from way back and to stop and feel the heartbeat of the earth through these majesties was soul enriching. To be in the land where part of my ancestors have roots gave an experience of connection on many levels. One I highly recommend.

Heading northeast we followed the path about one half mile then turned west before Connachan Lodge towards the Shaggie Burn. At this point we were just warming up as the cold wind was finally dying down. The previous days of hiking all day were starting to fray Lee's nerves and I knew I had to be extra careful what I said especially the way I used inflection. It had been this way from the time of construction on our business. I was too know Lee's non-verbal thoughts and I fell into the role without hesitation because I wanted to please. This was part of my coping behavior from abuses I had endured as a child. Right or wrong the programming on both sides were becoming more pronounced the longer we were together. It didn't help that, at this moment in time, both of us were tired and frustrated. Triggers on both sides were being exposed.

The role of victim in our generation wasn't tolerated, especially for women in the home and men in the workforce. If you had a job, and/or a stable home, then you were considered fortunate and thus had no right to complain. Add on top of that a religious upbringing and the dye was cast. I eased out of the religious life between sixteen and eighteen years old after one of the leaders in our church had me followed. It was by a friend that I trusted and she reported all my actions except for when I was home. It was heart breaking and it angered me. This was one of the things I took in deeply and flipped into break away freedom and addiction mode when I left home at eighteen.

Back on the trail Lee and I were now walking toward Monzie (pronounced MY-knee). We had gotten turned around and realized we were moving west when we needed to head northwest. So we cut through a field and found a dirt road that lead directly to Monzie. I knew when we were close and so did Lee because the energy slowed our pace.

As we approached the town the site of yellow caution tape was visible around the church graveyard. It was so old the headstones were tilting in on themselves and to their sides with heavy decaying. If this had been a modern cemetery it might have been different but these headstones were huge, granite with some standing six feet. In addition the ground was sinking in places. The energy felt off. Not light but heavy and somewhat dark.

     SHAMAN MELODIE MCBRIDE

It was around noon so we walked a little farther until we came upon a little white gate next to a lovely stream just off the path about twenty paces. We opened the unlocked gate and went through hoping to find a nice place by the stream to have lunch.

Not thinking, it directed us up a thinly wooded path along the creek that opened up to a large back yard with owners! There stood an older couple staring at us as we emerged. Both Lee and I were all over ourselves with apologies. The husband and wife, which were taking a break from gardening, said that the path was along the Shaggie Burn, as it is called, and all was well. They eased our minds about invading their privacy and wanted to know our story.

As I began to describe our journey I observed the posture of energy in this middle aged couple. The woman had a wide brimmed straw garden hat with her mid-length red grey locks tucked behind her ears. She also had gardening gloves to match her sundress that covered a thin figure. Her smile was radiant and welcoming. Her husband was tall, clean shaven with a medium build. His voice was pleasant and they both radiated health and vitality. They were in sync with the environment they had created. The Kelly green all around was astounding. It swallowed us up like an emerald gems clarity. It was bright, warm and flowing with peaceful energy. There was a greenhouse atrium that was all glass modified with white iron rod arches. It stood about fifty yards from their bright white renovated school house that was from around the early nineteen hundreds. A variety of trees, plants and flowers…everywhere. With the sound of the stream to synthesize it all surrounded by the warming sun.

Upon finishing our story, and stating that we had only wanted to have picnic lunch by the stream, Lee asked about the town of Monzie and its people. A sparkle lit up our gentleman host eyes and the legend of Kate began to flow from his being in a joyful manner.

Kate McFae (also known as Kate McNieven) was a healer and herbalist who was convicted as a witch in the sixteenth century. She was place in a barrel of tar, lit a fire and rolled downed Knock Hill into Monzie. Before she was so brutally murdered she put three curses on the village; first there would be no male children born in the Meyhouse

Manse (now known as The Old Manse of Monzie), second the pastors of Monzie Parish church would all go mad, and third Monzie castle would burn to the ground.

As I listened to this tall gentleman weave his tale, I began to imagine the events as they unfolded. It was easy because the area was still in the grips of the tale. There had been no male errs born in the Mayhouse, three pastors were said to go mad and the Monzie castle had burned down several times. Such energy being reinforced over and over again was blatantly evident. Plus the story that Kate had been tarred and feathered, placed in a barrel that was lit a fire and rolled down Knock hill towards Monzie was a reinforcement by the man's telling.

Trying to imagine the emotions Kate experienced by and from fellow human beings is unfathomable in the current era. On the other side the fear the perpetrators were inundated with in order to do this to another human being is gut wrenching. They truly must have believed she was not of this earth. In addition that she was hard to kill and to stay dead. The energy that has been reinforced has made the situation understandable but not comprehensible. The pain and anguish can only be imagined. The fact that fear promoted this behavior in the human psyche to be justifiable is something that, today, we still must be wary of in our society. Normalization of abuses in any civilization is an avenue to extinction.

After chit-chatting for a while longer we asked to eat our lunch beside their creek. The lovely couple agreed with proper hospitality and joyful smiles. As we sat and ate Lee and I knew we were not going to make it to the cave that day and we would hike back to the hotel. We waved goodbye to our hosts and verbally declared that the day was for Kate. Here's to Kate!

Turretbank was the road we took out of Monzie. It was lined with cup marked boulders with multiple large holes evident from some being removed. One can only imagine what the large stones would be used for as it wasn't something you could just throw in a bag. These were huge holes and the stones had to weigh several hundred pounds. There were also tall ancient trees that we took time to feel with our Reiki hands. To touch such magnificence placed my energy in such a happy space.

     SHAMAN MELODIE MCBRIDE

The weather was just right with a light breeze and every now and then you could hear a trickling stream in the background. So, so relaxing.

I must admit that I had partially disconnected from my hiking buddy's discomfort. That wasn't to last long though as Lee became vocal several miles from our nice creek side luncheon.

I did understand Lee's frustration. It had been three days of nothing but walking and climbing up and down paths and through frost laden fields. The look on Lee's face was 'I'm done'! I was hesitant when I said it but I still asked if everything was alright because I cared. I prepared myself for the onslaught as I had experienced many time before and to my disappointment this time was no different.

It's like the moment when a race car corners. You see the car lower and hug the road as it glides smoothly into the turn. This was Lee's way. The tone became cold and filled with direct energy that cut out exactly what was to happen from here forward. Calmly and precise like a surgeon. I knew I would be continuing this part of the journey alone. I was alright with it though because it was my vision that had promoted the trip in the first place. I had my role to play and so did Lee.

We agreed that Lee could go no further as almost forty miles in three days had taken its toll. Lee's body was sore and tired along with frayed nerves and emotional imbalance. There had to be a rebalancing for both and both agreed. Lee wanted to visit a rare mineral shop in town and pick up groceries. The amazing day of walking brought us along the backside of the huge Crieff Hydro estate and right to our back door.

When we arrived at the cabin that night I settled in and began to fix a nice dinner when I heard a guttural scream from Lee in the bathroom. I shut off the burned and ran to see what happened. There was all six feet of Lee standing on the toilet. Looking down I could see this huge black harry spider. I backed away and held my laughter. I grabbed a towel and threw it over the beast. There was a grunt as I watched Lee leap down right on top of the linen crushing the arachnid. Naked and now unafraid Lee wrapped up the kill and threw it in the corner. Yup I just lost it. I was laughing so hard the tears were flowing. Lee chuckled and got dressed as I closed the door and went back to making dinner.

As we sat down Lee was much better and relived the spider incident laughing during the telling. Lee cleaned up the kitchen and went to bed. I sat in the living room and mapped out a plan to hike into the highlands of Scotland alone.

CHAPTER 7

The Cave

EARLY THE NEXT morning I had my map, warm clothes and food for lunch. We went to town first to pick up fresh scallops for me to cook for dinner. Lee would get the accompanying vegetables in town later. Mid-morning, after it warmed a bit, Lee went with me in a taxi to drop me off on the path into the mountains. We drove east to Gilmerton and turned north on A822. After crossing an old stone arched bridge we stopped at a small sign that said foot path to Loch Tay. I would meet them back there at five o'clock that evening. It was go time for me and one step at a time was the best way to get there.

To say I was nervous wouldn't cover the emotions that were raging. The night before I had gone over the route I would take. I was still not one-hundred percent sure where the Druids cave was located. Laughing to myself, I wasn't sure I'd be able to find the cave at all but that wasn't going to stop me one iota. I had the map from town, the book on ley lines, plus the maps from the Innerpeffray library. The plan was to hike three miles to a foot path that went straight up a mountain and then cut back on a ridge to a valley that was on top of the mountain. I had gotten a good night's rest because trotting around the Scotland highlands for three days was starting to take its toll on my body but my endurance was high along with my adrenaline. I was determined to give it my all.

Waving goodbye to Lee as the taxi turned around and headed back to Crieff I began walking. The road was dirt and wide enough so two vehicles could squeeze by one another. There was a small white farm house with a stone fence on the back side now known as Newton. I could see a small older man standing in his back yard watching me as I walked around a corner and out of his site. I became clam. My senses opened and now I could connect with this natural environment.

The road slowly inclined and the day had a light breeze with the sun bringing warmth to the early morning. The day unfolded as I moved down the path where sheep were grazing in the shallow glens and small creeks trickled behind the sound they made. The air smell was fresh and stone fences lined the hills with precision edifice while the wind rustled the trees like a whisper. It gave me joyous chills.

I had timed my speed to pace a mile earlier in the trip so I knew when it was about three miles. I estimated it would take me six and a half hours. I passed a waterfall that would make a wonderful place for a snack on the way back. Further on I stopped and looked at a mountain with its narrow line running up its face. There was a thick group of conifers that matched those on the map. I double checked. This is it the one I'm going to climb! I say that because there wasn't one road up but three! Hence the reason for timing my pace. All of this planning came down to this…chaos. I felt it all through my being.

I took a deep breath and headed up the middle path but in order to get there I had to cut through a fenced pasture full of sheep. Trying not to disturb them very much as I opened and closed the squeaky metal gates. Sure of my destination but wary of the path forward. After passing through a bog of soft ground the climb became steeper. I had to walk across larger rocks now, then shale for about half mile. I could see nothing and was approaching the snow line. My body was shaking and I was sweating. Exhaustion was taking hold. I had to keep my wits about me so I sat on a boulder and asked the universe for a sign to guide me.

As I looked up I thought I saw movement. Looking closer in the prickle weeds I spotted a beautiful deep red headed grouse. It had seen me and looked at me as if it was waiting for me to notice its presence. 'Show me' I said. Then it flew to the edge of the ravine, landing it looked back at me. I followed. When I approached the bird it turned its head to the ravine. There was no cave. All I could see was a large old dead tree on the side of the corresponding mountain all alone. There were no other trees on that mountain at all. Then my messenger flew back to the trail again. I followed and when I look toward the top of the hill I saw that the clouds had parted to show the blue sky in the shape

     SHAMAN MELODIE MCBRIDE

of a smoke signal. Unusual to see the sky do this. It's more common to see this in cloud formations.

Covered with prickly seeds on my socks and feeling the burn of blisters on my boot laden feet I continued my ascent. My legs were a lot heavier now. It had been another mile. I was sweating pretty hard something that's unusual for me. As I approached the crest there was the sound of water. Stepping onto the flat plan there was a face starring back at me. My heart lightened for there it was, an ancient monolith, smiling at me. The same face that was in the pages of the ley line book. I had found it. With a mix of exuberance and exhaustion I dropped to my knees. There it was a huge man made cave of milky quartz and granite. I arose to investigate. To touch my reality. The water I could hear was from an underground stream flowing gently around the Druid's cave. The day was partly cloudy and my energy shifted wide open.

I spotted an alter about eight feet in front of the cave. I approached it and was going to touch it but pulled back. Something else had warranted my attention. Looking down the valley I could see the lone old tree. This was the tree from the legend that I had read in the ley line book months ago. This Scots pine story states that if a person breaks off one of its branches the person will die and the tree survive. The tree still stands as a tribute to the superstitions associated with its stories.

As I slowly made my way to the entrance of the cave there, on the ground to the right of the opening, was a dead white rabbit. There was no blood and the marks suggested that a large raptor had torn into the animals flesh. I know from the behavior of the hawks in my mountainous home that they will move a carcass to an area and save it for later. This appeared to be the case but the underlying question remains. Why here and why now? Transformation and/or creation would be my first impression. Death equals rebirth of self by extreme measures…chaos. In addition, the energy of the mountain suggested an influence to relationships. I would wait on these thoughts as my direction of mind was to enter the cave. So I gently moved the rabbit to the edge of the cave with a stick as not to contaminate the bird's future meal with my essence. I gave thanks for its purpose and sacrifice for the massage that was sure to unfold for me in the future. I smudged the cave and area with white sage.

Entering the cave I felt an energy that was akin to a magnetic field. If I moved off center I could feel an upward pull verses a downward pull positioning myself in the opposite corner of the cave. It was a small space that you could park a car into but the energy was immense. I knelt and reaching into my small rock pouch. It was black leather with buckskin fringe and had a buffalo nickel to fasten it. It had been hanging on my belt since the beginning of this quest and carried my power stones. I pulled out five small Satyaloka crystals. The crystals are blessed by Buddhist monks. Spiritual awakening and planetary consciousness is the energy they match. Digging a deep hole in the middle of the cave I buried them and proceeded to energize them with Reiki. I meditated to send healing energy through this nucleus and promote positive energy to our Mother Earth and all her inhabitants.

After completing the ceremony I photographed myself in front of the cave and around the cave to complete my research. I no longer felt exhaustion but elation. I was humbled at the magnificence the universe had not only allowed me to receive, but the energy I would hold within me for the rest of my life…and beyond.

The path down the mountain was a much easier go. My destination was a small outcrop with a little waterfall surrounded by tall trees that I had passed on my way up. It was there that I was heading to eat and rest before I hiked back to the prearranged meeting space with Lee. I was on schedule to make the rendezvous with my transport.

The afternoon was calm, peaceful and light. It was like floating in a dream and the sound of the water fall was sweet as I neared the cove. I sat down using a large trees trunk for a backstop. I had an apple, cheese and protein bar to regain my strength with cool water to wash it all down. While I was enjoying the moment of this huge accomplishment my mind began to wander back seven years ago when I had made the choice to live my life again. I took a deep breath and drifted into the past. Again.

As the sound of the water brought me into the present I realized I better get moving. I packed my gear and began my pace once again.

          SHAMAN MELODIE MCBRIDE

I felt so complete. Heading down the road I passed by the little white house and waved at the man who was outside working. Approaching the head of the trail I turned to look at the valley. This memory I wanted engrained with positive energy.

The taxi rounded the corner and stopped. The door opened to a look on Lees face that was relief and excitement combined. I climbed in and as the taxi turned around the drivers relief was also visible. In a calm voice I stated I had found the Druids cave. Lee smiled and said 'I knew you would but now I have something to show you back in town'. I was surprised and I could've felt deflated but I was too much in the energy of victory, humility and yes exhaustion. On to town.

Lee began rambling about getting money from the hole in the wall i.e. ATM, because the rock shop was going to close and a purchase needed to be made. Lee had spent the day running errands and getting chatty with the locals. That was the conversation all the way back to town. The taxi dropped us off at the money machine where Lee withdrew some cash. We then walked up the street to the rare minerals shop where a sweet little older lady was patiently waiting. She greeted us and offered us tea which I thought was strange since it was her closing time. Lee looked at her and winked as if to say now. With that this polite little lady picked up the phone and made a call. The other end was to a gentleman named David that lived over the shop. She asked him to come downstairs to meet us. To my utter surprise the man that showed up was none other than David Cowan the author of the Ley Line book I had been following this whole time. I was speechless! I mean how humbling that the universe could be so allowing, so unpredictably amazing. I really could not find the words to express how grateful I was to be in this moment in time.

I asked David to sign my book, which he was happy to do, and we sat, had a cup of tea and spoke of the profound synchronicities in our universe. I could hear the shop owner ask Lee if I was always this quiet. Lee's response was of astonishment for this had not been something that had been witness ever throughout our relationship. A smile appeared on all our faces. The time had come to head back to the cabin as the next day we would leave the highlands. Truth be known I pinched myself several times to make sure all of it was real. After I returned home I would email David a picture I took of the cave since he hadn't seen it for twenty years. That which connects us holds what compels us.

CHAPTER 8

Art the back to Ireland

I SLEPT WELL, VERY well that night and awoke to a beautiful day and Lees smiling face. We had packed up our stuff the night before along with having a fabulous dinner, if I do say so myself. All we had to do was finish our breakfast and call the taxi to take us to train station.

Leaving Crieff was a mixture of energies for me. I had accomplished an astounding feat yet I felt as if it was an ordinary occurrence. Throughout all the strife, and synchronicity, the end was unpredictable but balanced. I knew the universe had taken what I manifested and given me this astounding sense of purpose. Staying in the moment with my thoughts and placing my actions bit-by-bit had given rise to calm. My soul was calm and I knew in that moment that I was connected. I was at peace. I had truly not experienced such an energy before and the astonishment was and is liberating.

Back in Glasgow we were supposed to check into the Premier Inn hotel on Argyle Street but because we were a day behind we cancelled. Instead we decided to walk to the museum. So we stopped at a shop along the way and grabbed a protein bar, water and some nuts to snack on as we walked. Of course it didn't seem that far on the map but the walk in downtown Glasgow was worth it. The architecture was amazing on St Vincent and Argyll Street as we hiked (again) to our destination the Kelvingrove.

The Kelvingrove museum is in an old castle. The original Kelvingrove Museum opened in the latter half of the nineteenth century. It was housed in an enlarged eighteenth century mansion called Kelvingrove House. It is made of beautiful red sandstone and was originally opened in 1901 for the Glasgow International Exhibition.

We realized that in order to spend the time we'd like in the museum we would have to get a taxi to the airport. Agreeing to that made Lee and I take ease so we could spend the afternoon getting through the exhibits.

Entering the front door the space opened. There was a pipe organ that was the center piece of the main floor but my attention was absorbed by the marble. The columns, stairs, floors, it all was so elegant and structured. The ceiling was cupped with recessed wooden square panels to move the sound. It felt like a time capsule. One that would exhibit art for the sake of history, melancholy and elation with a higher disconnect that pushed one to awaken familiar energies of the ancestors.

Lee had located a map of the museum and because we were to meet Mattie at the airport our time was directed toward the early Celtic tribal findings and paintings from the masters. Then if we had time we would work our way down from the top floor down.

Climbing the crisp marble stairs I could see the enclosed rooms of the first floor which was actually the top floor since the ground floor was the entrance. The lower ground was where the café and shops were located. First we went to the Scottish first people's exhibit then the conflict and consequence and finally we went to the East side where the hanging art was featured. This area also has security guards and when I looked at the paintings floating on the walls I could see why.

It began with Rembrandt and Monet, Gauguin and Renoir then Titian and Salvador Dali. The landscapes moved me so much so that I didn't realize I was moving closer. The guards then reminded me of my proximity. I looked at the two security men and stated I was so enthralled I just wasn't paying attention. They acknowledged it happens often and I proceeded back to my dream state of admiration. I must say that the energy in Claude Monet's landscapes drew me in. The strokes had a beautiful rhythm. It reminded me of the classes I took with my Mother as a youth and clear into high school. Nature has always drawn me into its fold. I was in my happy place when Lee reminded me of our time restraints. I begrudgingly tore myself away as we headed back down the stairs to catch a taxi to the airport.

     SHAMAN MELODIE MCBRIDE

Mattie was waiting for us at the terminal as we embraced and began our rendition of the past few day's events. He was awestruck and fascinated but still in disbelief of how it all unfolded. So was I. Still struck by the humbling of my spirit. The clam, the peace within my soul and to end the Scottish visit in the presence of such masters of art. I just felt so truly blessed. I give gratitude for the artist.

As we landed in Belfast we met Maggie at the terminal. Her flight from Dublin had arrived around the same time as ours 9:30 PM. Mattie went to get the car out of parking while we gathered our bags from the carousel and we were off to Mattie's. That evening we repacked again to head for the Northern coast in the morning. That's all the info Lee and I had been given. Mattie had been conversing with Maggie the past few days. Our giddy host had come up with a new plan since Lee and I took an extra day in Crieff.

The next morning our cohorts were excited about their secret plans. Mattie had fun taunting me as I loved surprises of this type and we were enjoying the banter between us. While Lee was much more cautious and reserved. That attitude ended though when we began to drive through the beautiful countryside. We stopped by some church graveyards to search for our family names. Lee found some and I found some on my Mother's side. There was another on the coast Mattie knew of that might contain my surname of McBride. Everything on the checklist for our trip was almost done.

The day was flowing along nicely when we came to our first stop at Glenveagh Castle and gardens. How could I go to Ireland and not visit a castle? Right? The castle was part of the Glenveagh National Park. Located in the heart of county Donegal, Ireland. Glenveagh mansion was castellated in 1870. The twenty-seven acre gardens are the centerpiece for the National Park. They have a huge variety of trees and flowers but I fancied the pristine herb garden. The smell sucks you in and holds you captive. Perma-grin set in as I was absorbed by the green. We were all happy and having a good time. We went through the castle and then the gardens. Taking photos by the garden statues did cause some interesting poses with tons of laughter. Al in all a great time was had.

When we reached the Atlantic coast Maggie had made reservations for us at a B&B named the Ostan Gweedore Hotel where a nice little elderly lady welcomed us with kindness and grace. The room was adorned with handmade lace doylies and fresh white linens. The smell was of the ocean and old coal. The view from our window was serene. The ocean was wild and I liked this. It was in the background as the owner told us of the buildings history. It was built in 1841 by Sir George Hill a wealthy landlord who developed Gweedore. The little lady relayed the story quickly as to not be too foreboding. It was centered around the landlord and his slow impacts that accelerated the famine and emigration. Although Hill did try to help the poor eventually it was deemed that his effects on the area almost led to the demise of the only area left that spoke Gaeltacht. The loss from the famine in her family, along with others, were displayed on the lobby walls. Gently she eased us back into the beauty of the area with the offer of a terraced meal by the sea. The kindness in the Irish is as fierce as their devotion to the land.

We had a lovely dinner at the Seaview restaurant. The tables were covered with white linen and set with silver utensils'. There were candles and the meal was served on elegant porcelain china. Mattie was getting more anxious to reveal a surprise for us so we all loaded into the gumdrop car and headed into the countryside.

After about twenty minutes Mattie became a little concerned over the route he was taking. After all this is from memory and it was going to be dark soon. Then we came upon a sign. A large red sigh that said Leo's home of Clannad and Enya BIA & CEOL 1st right after Crolly Bridge 3K. 'What? Enya's family establishment? Groovy!' was my response. 'We have to have a picture by the sigh while it's still light' I said. Lee and I stood on either end while Maggie snapped the shot and then we were off again. Ten minutes later we pulled into a parking area behind a two story white building. We entered through a side door to see families and Clannad playing an Irish jig.

Leo, come to find out, was Enya's father and Mattie was taking us to show us what a family tavern in Ireland really was all about. This included Guinness for everyone except me. I had soda water. I had done

     SHAMAN MELODIE MCBRIDE

my bit with alcohol in my twenties and wasn't about to go down that road ever again. We sat at a table that was under one of Enya's platinum records and listened to the music. We were joking and laughing enjoying the ambiance when the music stopped and the bands leader asked if anyone in the audience would like to sing with them. I didn't think anything about it until Maggie burst out my name and pointed at me! I was shocked and politely refused but they were determined so I went up there and introduced myself. The lead singer asked me to pick any song and I went blank completely blank. Eventually they picked a song and I sang along. I don't remember what the songs title was but I had a great time! Enjoying the conversation and fun filled atmosphere we stayed for a while longer. The families had finished their meals and ushered all out the door. We then felt it was time for us to drive back to the B&B. What a treasure this gift from our new Irish friend.

The day began with the sound of seabirds and ocean waves. Already packed we had a lite breakfast and headed to the seashore. Bad Eddie boat on the Bunbeg beach could be seen from our rooms. The boat had been shipwreck and washed ashore in nineteen seventy. It was sunny and cool but didn't stop us from pictures around the wreck and collecting Irish glass and seashells among the white sand. After building a sandcastle that fell apart we decided to have a little picnic in the Druid's restaurant that we spied as we were playing in the sand. It was filling which was fine because the adventure for the day had just begun.

Piling into the red gingerbread man's button we drove to the Donegal cemetery. There I found the McBride's. A large area of the graveyard was filled with my relatives. All graves covered with crystal white granite gravel. Profound that I who lived and loved in the mountains had lineage from the sea. There were also countless unmarked graves. Signs of the past atrocities still relevant in the future. As the innkeeper said, 'The fear of war is great'.

We arrived back at Mattie's late. Tomorrow would be our last day in Ireland and my emotions were mixed.

CHAPTER 9

The Wall

LEE AND I took some time to pack since all that we had sent now had to fit in our suitcases. Lee would jump on top of the cases while I zipped. It was the morning workout.

The day's plan was full and we were off to Belfast to shop. Mattie actually liked shopping so he guided us to the shops after we dropped off our disposable cameras to be developed. Belfast was full of beautiful architecture and colorful people from all over the world. We went to several Celtic novelty stores where items were bought that represented the Irish craftsman in woven metal and artesian delights.

Maggie had wanted us to see an old building downtown that had an old vaudeville mid-twenties theme with tall green marble pillars and high glass ceilings. It was the Merchant Hotel and it was stunning. A five star hotel in the historic Cathedral Quarter where we were shopping. A late lunch/ early dinner was a sit down at a nice place. While eating Mattie had asked me to teach the Vipassana meditation techniques I had learned to his class that night. I was honored and agreed.

Maggie, Lee and I attended Mattie's class at Queen's University that evening. I had brought the Tibetan bells to balance the energy in the classroom so teaching a different form of meditation to the students would fit nicely into this energy. All four of us have experience in the healing fields so everyone played a part teaching the students about positive healing vibrations in and of the body. The lessons were well received and we all learned something unique to self in the process. There was another subject had come to light during the class. That of the Irish past so afterword the four of us walked to a small coffee shop to talk.

The conversation moved into the long war between Brittan and Ireland. The North Unionists Protestants' against the Irish Catholics in the rest of the county. Mattie stated that sometimes he had a challenging time communicating to his young students the value in the overall energy that was created. I had felt his frustration so much so that in the moment I had a waking vision. Communication was the focal point. I had a Lapis pendant that was small I carried with me to reinforce my vocal energy. I knew it would help Mattie. Lee knew how much it meant to me. I took it off and gave it to Mattie, 'and when you have learned what you need to from it pass it on' I said. The surprise on Lee and Maggie's faces was priceless as tears filled their eyes. Mattie on the other hand had tears in his eyes and thanked me through a lump in his throat. Then he said let me show you something. We loaded into the gumdrop and headed to the wall.

Now understand that the British military had only been gone for six months and violence was still prevalent. One part of the wall Mattie took us was the memorial of Bobby Sands who died on a hunger strike at HM Prison maze in Northern Ireland on May 5, 1981. I reminisced hearing this on the news as it was my senior high school graduation that month. As we were standing there a Molotov cocktail came flying over the tops of our heads smashing into the netted fence leaving a bright petrol orange fire on the wall in the dark next to us. Time to go! As we drove Mattie told us of the death mile where they still had shootings every night.

It was dark so we attempted to get to the British side. We found only one gate was open to the protestant side which surprised even Mattie. He wanted to show us the murals on the unionists' side which was dangerous especially for him. If as an Irish man he was caught there past curfew he could be detained or shot. Once across the barrier I saw militants' murals. It looked so different from the Irish catholic side. One mourned its dead and the other celebrated its killing ability. Once the car was noticed guns began to appear from the darkness. This was frontline reality that Mattie wanted us to see and understand. An emotion all too familiar to a man and his people who love the sea. Mattie was getting more anxious so we made a beeline out of there.

To finish the night, like all this wasn't enough, we drove past the peace wall. Also called the hero's wall. It celebrated those who forged an alliance of peace and drafted the Good Friday agreement.

Whoa the line a man has made
Your world goods may cross the woven knot
The drum, the strum, the wood click
Whoa the line man placed solid
Paint the unity slashing power…hope
Whoa the line that cuts the green
Is this sacrificed image of man or
Beast as pressed as both
Power masked played the long grief game
Whoa the bog sorrow bound south
To dark blind complicity
Green of Spring finds life light
Grow, thrive, renaissance soul
Shaman Melodie McBride

The next morning we had time for a late breakfast and then headed to the airport. Our flight left in the late afternoon which gave Lee and I time to reflect before boarding. I took my journal with me and once we were boarded and in the air I began to write. I wrote for almost the entire trip to the US. Lee was somewhat in another place and looked at me coldly stating I had changed. I didn't respond but that statement would manifest into the Druid cave's white rabbit and chaos was to follow.

I am not from Ireland my ancestors were though. They migrated to the US during the great potato famine.

You have worked to get to the place you stand. Stand tall, stand firm, stand in the whole entire of your space. If the box has solid sides evolution of self will experience only what brought you to the inside of this space. Step outside…the view is the magnificence of your unbound…

 SHAMAN MELODIE MCBRIDE

CLOSING

Analysis of the steps that moved into the cycle toward chaos and back. Plus energy that was created to move forward into the next venture.

1. Energy moved forward at a rapid pace once the decision was made to find the cave.
2. Obstacles began when starting out and we had to turn around to get glasses.
3. Sickness of body. Plugged and then released. Attributed to how fast the flow was moving and energies causing a push me pull me affect.
4. The unmanned train station arrangements made by another who had different energy caused difficulties in relationship expectations.
5. Struggle through ignorance (mind state) some of which could not be prepared for because of the unknown factors involved.
6. Gratitude and silence in victory like meditative awakening.
7. Shared animosity on flight home to US.

These steps are a recognition in the cycle (entire trip) and the choices made to relieve or change the outcome. Taking into account that which is reinforced from the cosmos, programmed upbringing and the environments in which it all took place. We will continue these analogies throughout the series tying them together in the last book. Keeping it simple is the first step. We will expand because we evolve.

This venture is based on a true story although names were changed. The interpretation may differ from others account. The references to places and historical sites can be found through websites along with transportation hubs. Because this is an event that is from the turn of the century some sources may be obsolete.